BREAST CANCER DIET FOR NEWLY DIAGNOSED

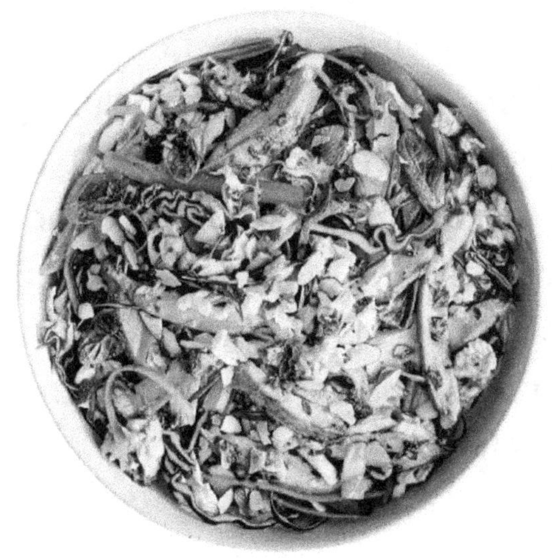

Irresistible Anti-Cancer Eats for Healing Shielding and Revitalising Your Wellness

Vera V. Janson

GAIN ACCESS TO MORE BOOK FROM ME

ABOUT THE AUTHOR

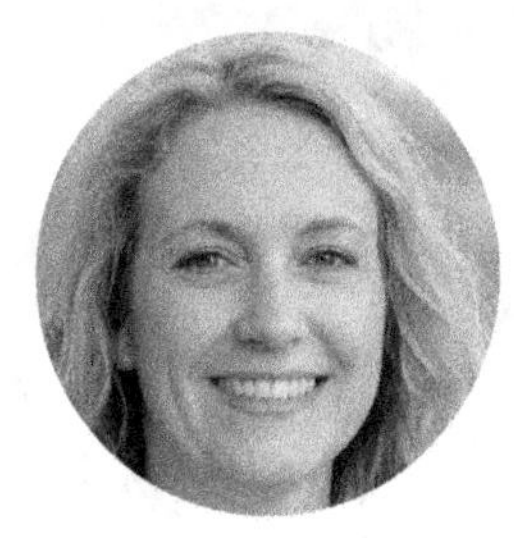

Vera V. Janson is an author specialising in healthy cooking. She has written several cookbooks filled with recipes for delicious and nutritious meals. Her work has helped many people find healthy alternatives to traditional dishes.

SPECIAL BONUS

Get Free 6 Weekly Meal Planner

TABLE OF CONTENT

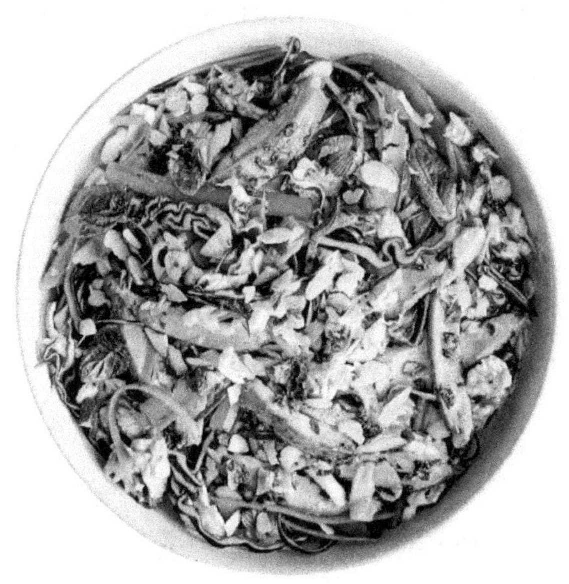

INTRODUCTION

This cookbook serves as a source of food and empowerment for those suffering breast cancer. Discover a culinary guide designed specifically for newly diagnosed patients, including not only recipes but also a road map to well-being. Each meal exemplifies the marriage of flavour and health, meticulously prepared to meet the individual nutritional requirements of patients undergoing treatment. Beyond the kitchen, this cookbook acts as a guide, offering insights into nutrition's transformative power.

It's more than just the **Ingredients**; it's a story of resilience, where the dish serves as a source of strength. Whether it's the vivid colours of antioxidant-rich fruits or the comforting warmth of nourishing soups, each recipe contributes to a better, tastier tomorrow. Embrace this cookbook as a companion.

Breast cancer is a complex disease that starts in the cells of the breast. It can affect both men and women, but it is significantly more prevalent in women. Understanding the many types, causes, symptoms, and prevention strategies is critical in the fight against breast cancer.

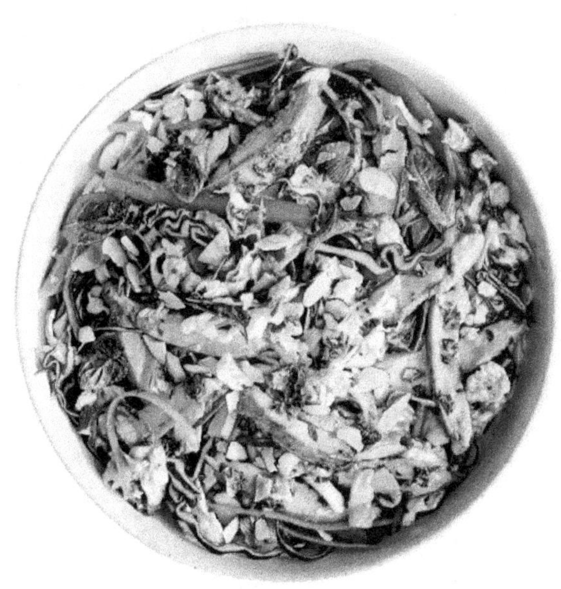

CHAPTER 1

Type of Breast Cancer

Breast cancer is classified into subtypes based on the individual cells affected. The two main types of breast cancer are non-invasive (in situ) and invasive. Non-invasive kinds include ductal carcinoma in situ (DCIS), in which abnormal cells are discovered in the lining of a breast duct but have not spread to adjacent tissues. Invasive breast cancer, on the other hand, penetrates surrounding healthy tissues and can be further classified into other histological categories, such as invasive ductal carcinoma and Invasive lobular cancer.

Causes of Breast Cancer

Breast cancer is caused by a combination of risk factors, but the specific reason remains unknown. Age, gender, and genetics have important factors. Women over the age of 50 are more likely to develop breast cancer, and having close relatives with the disease increases vulnerability. The existence of particular gene mutations, such as BRCA1 and BRCA2, is associated to an increased risk of developing breast cancer. Hormonal factors, oestrogen exposure, reproductive history, and certain lifestyle choices such as obesity and alcohol intake all contribute to the risk.

Symptoms of Breast Cancer

Early detection of breast cancer relies on recognising its signs. Common symptoms include the existence of a lump or thickening in the breast, changes in the size, shape, or appearance of the breast, and inexplicable discomfort or tenderness. Skin changes such as redness, dimpling, or puckering should be observed. Other than breast milk, discharge from the nipple and changes in nipple position can both be signs of breast cancer. Regular self-examinations and mammograms are critical for spotting these symptoms early, increasing the likelihood of successful treatment.

Preventive measures can dramatically reduce the risk of breast cancer. Regular physical activity helps to maintain a healthy weight and lowers oestrogen levels, which contributes to breast cancer prevention. A well-balanced diet high in fruits, vegetables, and whole grains contains important nutrients and antioxidants. Limiting alcohol consumption and avoiding smoke are important protective measures.

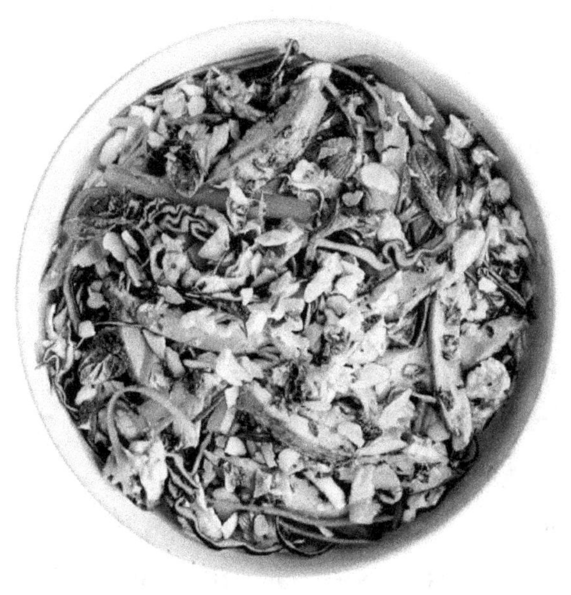

CHAPTER 2

A well-balanced and nutrient-dense diet is essential for people battling breast cancer because it promotes overall health and aids in the management of treatment side effects. While nutritional requirements vary depending on individual circumstances, there are broad guidelines for what foods to include and avoid in a breast cancer disease diet.

Foods to Include:

1. Incorporate colourful fruits and veggies into your diet. These foods are high in antioxidants, vitamins, and minerals, which promote general health. Berries, leafy greens, citrus fruits, and cruciferous vegetables (such as broccoli) are especially healthy.

A well-balanced and nutrient-rich diet is crucial for individuals navigating breast cancer, supporting overall health and aiding in the management of treatment side effects. While nutritional needs may vary based on individual circumstances, there are general guidelines on foods to include and avoid in a breast cancer disease diet.

2. Lean Proteins:

Choose lean protein sources such as chicken, fish, beans, and lentils. Protein is necessary for tissue repair and immunological function. Fish, particularly fatty fish such as salmon, contain omega-3 fatty acids, which are anti-inflammatory.

3.   Whole Grains:

Choose whole grains over refined grains to get more fibre and minerals. Brown rice, quinoa, whole wheat, and oats are great options. Fibre assists digestion and promotes a healthy weight.

4. Healthy Fats:

Consume healthy fats in moderation, such as avocados, nuts, seeds, and olive oil. These fats contain necessary fatty acids and can promote general health.

5. Dairy or Dairy Alternatives:

Calcium is essential for bone health, and dairy or fortified dairy products are excellent sources. To limit your calorie intake, go for low-fat or non-fat options.

6. Hydration:

Stay hydrated by drinking plenty of water. Proper hydration is critical for general health and can help control adverse effects from treatments such as chemotherapy.

Foods to Limit

1. Processed and Red Meat:

Limit your consumption of processed meats, such as sausages and bacon, as well as red meat. High consumption of these foods has been linked to an elevated risk of certain malignancies.

2. Sugary Foods and Beverages:

Reduce your intake of sugary foods and drinks. High sugar consumption can cause weight gain and inflammation. When you have a sweet need, opt for natural sweeteners such as honey or fruits.

3. Alcohol:

Limit your alcohol consumption, as it has been related to an increased risk of breast cancer. If you choose to drink, do so moderately.

4. Highly Processed Foods:

Limit your intake of highly processed and refined foods. These frequently contain additional sugars, harmful fats, and lack the nutritional benefits of entire meals.

5. Saturated and Trans Fats:

Reduce your intake of saturated and trans fats by avoiding fried foods, pastries, and certain margarines. These fats can promote inflammation and have a negative influence on general health.

6. Caffeine:

While data into caffeine's effects on breast cancer is ambiguous, some people may choose to reduce their caffeine intake. It is advisable to discuss personal preferences with healthcare practitioners.

Customizing the Diet

Individual nutritional requirements during breast cancer therapy may vary, and it is critical to tailor the diet to unique conditions. Some people may notice changes in taste, appetite, or trouble swallowing, prompting dietary changes. Consulting with a licenced dietician or nutritionist can provide personalised advice and assist with any issues.

Finally, for people dealing with breast cancer, eating a well-balanced and nutritious diet is critical to their overall health. Nutrient-dense foods can help the body during treatment and recovery, leading to better health and a higher quality of life. Always seek personalised advice from healthcare specialists regarding individual health conditions and treatment approaches.

1. Nutritional Support:

Following a breast cancer disease diet ensures that the body gets enough nutrients, vitamins, and minerals. Adequate diet promotes general health and allows the body to deal with the physical demands of cancer therapy.

2. Immune System Enhancement:

A well-balanced diet helps to boost the immune system. This is critical during breast cancer therapy because a strong immune response helps the body fight off infections and promotes speedier healing.

3. Weight Management:

Maintaining a healthy weight is linked to improved results in breast cancer treatment. A well-balanced diet high in whole foods and low in processed and sugary foods aids in weight management and lowers the risk of obesity-related problems.

4. Inflammation Reduction

Many items in a breast cancer diet, including fruits, vegetables, and omega-3 fatty acids, are anti-inflammatory. This can be especially useful for reducing treatment-related inflammation and promoting the body's healing process.

5. Energy and stamina:

The appropriate combination of carbs, proteins, and fats gives long-lasting energy, reducing weariness that is common throughout cancer treatments. This supports daily activities and contributes to a higher quality of life.

6. Bone Health:

Certain breast cancer medications may have an influence on bone health. Adequate calcium and vitamin D intake, which can be found in dairy or fortified foods, helps to maintain strong and healthy bones.

7. Digestive Health:

A breast cancer diet high in fibre from fruits, vegetables, and whole grains improves digestive health. This is especially crucial for addressing the potential gastrointestinal adverse effects of cancer therapy.

8. Emotional Wellbeing:

Nourishing the body with nutritious foods can improve mental and emotional well-being. It gives you a sense of control and empowerment during a difficult period, which contributes to a more optimistic attitude.

9. Hydration and Detoxification:
Staying hydrated helps the body's natural detoxification processes. Proper hydration is critical for cleaning out toxins and maintaining normal organ function, which is especially important during cancer treatment.

10. Support for Treatment Side Effects:
Some foods, such as ginger and peppermint, may help relieve nausea and stomach difficulties caused by certain cancer therapies. A breast cancer diet tailored to individual needs can help patients manage treatment side effects more effectively.

11. Lowered Risk of Recurrence:
While no diet may ensure prevention, a good diet may help to lower the chance of breast cancer recurrence. Following dietary guidelines after treatment can help maintain long-term health and well-being.

12. Lifestyle Habits:
Adopting a breast cancer illness diet is frequently associated with the promotion of other

healthy lifestyle practices. This includes regular physical activity, stress management, and avoiding tobacco use, all of which contribute to a well-rounded approach to health.

Individuals who choose a breast cancer disease diet empower themselves to take an active role in their treatment process. Dietary choices should be tailored to individual health circumstances, treatment regimens, and preferences. Consulting with healthcare specialists, including registered dieticians, ensures that nutrition is tailored to the specific needs of each breast cancer patient.

1. Colourful Berries:
   Berries such as blueberries, strawberries, and raspberries are high in antioxidants, which help reduce inflammation and promote general health.

2) Cruciferous Vegetables:
   Combine broccoli, cauliflower, Brussels sprouts, and kale. These veggies include chemicals that have been linked to a lower cancer risk.

3. Leafy Greens: Spinach, kale, and Swiss chard include critical vitamins, minerals, and antioxidants that promote general health.

4. Lean Protein Sources:

Choose skinless poultry, fish, beans, lentils, and tofu. These are high-quality protein sources that are low in saturated fat.

5. Fatty fish:

Salmon, mackerel, and sardines contain omega-3 fatty acids, which have anti-inflammatory qualities.

6. Whole Grain:

Brown rice, quinoa, oats, and whole wheat are good sources of fibre, vitamins, and minerals.

7. Nuts and Seeds: Almonds, walnuts, chia seeds, and flaxseeds contain beneficial fats and nutrients.

8. Avocado:

Avocado is a nutrient-dense fruit high in beneficial monounsaturated fats and vitamins.

9. Dairy or Fortified substitutes: Ensure appropriate calcium intake from sources like low-fat dairy, almond milk, or other fortified substitutes.

10. Colourful Vegetables:

Include a variety of vegetables, such as carrots, bell peppers, and sweet potatoes, for a wide spectrum of vitamins and antioxidants.

11. Turmeric:

This spice contains curcumin, which is known for its anti-inflammatory qualities. Consult a healthcare expert before using turmeric in cooking or taking turmeric supplements.

12. Garlic:

Garlic includes sulphur compounds, which may have anticancer effects. Add it to meals for flavour and probable health benefits.

13. Ginger:

Ginger, which is well-known for its anti-nausea properties, can help manage treatment-related symptoms. Use it in cooking or to make tea.

14. Green Tea:

Green tea contains several antioxidants, including catechism, which may have cancer-fighting qualities.

15. Beans and legumes:

Lentils, chickpeas, and black beans are rich in plant-based protein and fibre.

16. Low-Sugar Fruits:
Choose fruits such as apples, pears, and berries for natural sweetness without added sugar.

17. Tomatoes:
Tomatoes contain lycopene, a potent antioxidant. Cooking tomatoes increases the absorption of lycopene.

18. Use whole wheat or alternate grain pasta for more fibre and minerals.

19. Olive oil:
Extra virgin olive oil is a healthy fat alternative for cooking and topping salads.

20. Herbs and Spices: Use herbs and spices like cilantro, parsley, thyme, and rosemary to boost flavour without adding too much salt.

Consult healthcare specialists, especially qualified dieticians, for personalised recommendations based on particular health circumstances.

CHAPTER 3

BREAKFAST

1. Berry and Greek Yoghurt Parfait

Ingredients

- One cup of Greek yoghurt.

- Add 1/2 cup mixed berries (strawberries, blueberries, raspberries) and 2 tbsp. granola.

- One teaspoon of honey.

Preparation:

- In a glass or dish, combine the Greek yoghurt, mixed berries, and granola.

- Drizzle the honey on top.

- Nutritive Value:

- This meal is well-balanced thanks to protein-rich Greek yoghurt, antioxidants from berries, and fibre in granola.

- Cook Time:

- Five minutes.

2. Avocado and Poached Egg Toast

Ingredients

- 1 slice whole grain bread - 1/2 ripe avocado (mashed)
- One poached egg.
- Add salt and pepper to taste

- **Preparation**:

- Toast the bread, then put mashed avocado on top.
- Add a poached egg to the avocado.
- Season with salt and pepper.
- Nutritional Value: - Avocado provides healthy fats, eggs provide protein, and whole grain bread contains fibre.
- Cook Time:
- 10 minutes

3. Quinoa and Mixed Berry Breakfast: Bowl

Ingredients:

- Use 1/2 cup cooked quinoa and 1/2 cup mixed berries.
- One tablespoon of sliced almonds.
- One teaspoon of honey.
- **Preparation**:
- In a bowl, combine the quinoa, mixed berries, and sliced almonds.
- Drizzle honey on top.
- Nutritional Value: - Quinoa gives protein, berries supply antioxidants, and almonds contribute healthy fats.
- Cooking time: 15 minutes, including quinoa cooking time.

4. Spinach and Feta Omelette

Ingredients:

- 2 beaten eggs

- 1 cup freshly chopped spinach.

- Two tablespoons of feta cheese.

- Add salt and pepper to taste

- **Preparation**:

- In a pan, cook the chopped spinach until wilted.

- Pour the beaten eggs over the spinach, sprinkle with feta, and simmer until set.

- Season with salt and pepper.

- Nutritional Value: - Eggs provide protein, spinach contains iron, and feta contains calcium.

- Cooking Time: 10 minutes

5. Chia Seed Pudding with Mango

Ingredients:

- Three tablespoons of chia seeds
- One cup almond milk.
- Add 1/2 teaspoon vanilla extract and 1/2 cup cubed mango.

Preparation:

- Combine chia seeds, almond milk, and vanilla essence in a bowl.
- Refrigerate overnight.
- Prior to serving, top with chopped mango.
- Nutritive Value:
- Chia seeds provide omega-3 fatty acids, while mango contains vitamins.
- Cooking Time: - 5 minutes (with overnight refrigeration)

6. Whole Grain Pancakes with Berries

Ingredients

- Use 1/2 cup whole wheat flour and 1/2 cup milk.
- Use 1 egg and 1/2 teaspoon baking powder.
- Mixed berries for topping.

Preparation:

- Combine the flour, milk, egg, and baking powder to produce pancake batter.
- Cook the pancakes on a griddle.
- Garnish with mixed berries.
- Nutritive Value:
- Whole wheat fibre, egg protein, and antioxidant-rich berries.
- Cooking time: 15 minutes.

7. Yoghurt and Fruit Smoothie Bowl

Ingredients

- 1 cup plain yoghurt.

- Half a banana

- -1/2 cup frozen mixed berries

- One tablespoon almond butter

- **Preparation**:

- Combine the yoghurt, banana, berries, and almond butter until smooth.

- Transfer to a bowl and, if desired, top with additional Ingredients.

- Nutritional Value: Contains probiotics from yoghurt, potassium from banana, and antioxidants from berries.

- Cooking Time: - 5 minutes

8. Smoked Salmon and Cream Cheese Bagel

- **Ingredients**:

- 1 whole grain bagel

- 2 tablespoons cream cheese

- 2 slices of smoked salmon

- Garnish with capers and fresh dill

- **Preparation**:

- Toast the bagel and spread cream cheese on both sides.

- Top with smoked salmon and garnish with capers and fresh dill.

- Nutritional value

- Omega-3 fatty acids from salmon and whole grains are high in fibre.

- Cooking Times:

- 10 Minutes

9. Peanut Butter and Banana Overnight Oats

Ingredients:

- 1/2 cup rolled oats and 1/2 cup milk.
- One spoonful peanut butter.
- 1/2 banana, cut

- **Preparation**:

- Combine oats, milk, and peanut butter in a container.

- Refrigerate overnight and garnish with sliced banana before serving.

- Nutritional Value: Contains protein from peanut butter, fibre from oats, and potassium from banana.

- Cooking Time: - 5 minutes (with overnight refrigeration)

10. Egg and Vegetable Breakfast: Wrap

Ingredients:

- One whole wheat tortilla.

- Two scrambled eggs.

- Sauté spinach, tomatoes, and bell peppers. Add 1 tablespoon feta cheese.

- Preparation:

- Fill each tortilla with scrambled eggs, sautéed veggies, and feta.

- Roll into a wrap and fasten with a toothpick, if necessary.

- Nutritive Value:

- Eggs provide protein, vegetables provide fibre, and feta contains calcium.

- Cook Time:

- 15 minutes (including vegetables sauté).

LUNCH

1. Quinoa Salad with Grilled Chicken

Ingredients:

- 1 cup cooked quinoa

- 4 ounces sliced grilled chicken breast

- 1 cup halved cherry tomatoes

- 1/2 diced cucumber.

- 1/4 cup crumbled feta cheese.

- Two teaspoons of olive oil.

- Add lemon juice, salt, and pepper to taste.

  Prepare:

- In a bowl, combine the quinoa, grilled chicken, tomatoes, cucumber, and feta.

- Drizzle with olive oil, then add lemon juice, salt, and pepper. Toss lightly.

- Nutritive Value:

- Chicken provides protein, quinoa and vegetables provide fibre, and olive oil provides healthy fat.
- Cooking Time: 20 minutes (including quinoa cooking time).

2. Salmon and Quinoa Stuffed Bell Peppers

Ingredients:

- 2 halved bell peppers
- 6 ounces cooked and flaked salmon
- 1 cup cooked quinoa
- 1/2 cup diced cherry tomatoes.
- 1/4 cup finely chopped red onion.
- Fresh herbs (parsley or dill)
- Salt and pepper to taste

- Preparation

- Preheat the oven to 375°F (190° C).

- Combine the flakes salmon, quinoa, tomatoes, red onion, and herbs.

- Stuff bell pepper halves with the mixture and bake until they are soft.

- Nutritive Value:

- Salmon provides omega-3 fatty acids, quinoa contains protein, and vegetables provide vitamins.

- Cooking Time: 30 minutes

3. Vegetarian Chickpea Stir-Fry

Ingredients:

- One cup cooked chickpeas.

- Mix vegetables (broccoli, bell peppers, snap peas) - Add 1 tablespoon soy sauce

- One tablespoon of sesame oil.

- 1 clove garlic, minced

- 1 teaspoon grated ginger.

- **Preparation**:

- In a wok or pan, cook mixed vegetables, chickpeas, garlic, and ginger in sesame oil.

- Add the soy sauce and simmer until the vegetables are tender-crisp.

- Nutritive Value:

- Chickpeas provide plant-based protein, veggies contain fibre, and sesame oil contains healthful fats.

- Cooking time: 15 minutes.

4. Turkey and Quinoa Stuffed Zucchini

Ingredients:

Ingredients: 2 halved zucchinis and 8 ounces cooked ground turkey.

- One cup cooked quinoa.

- 1/2 cup black beans (drained and rinsed)

-1/2 cup salsa

- 1 teaspoon of cumin, chilli powder, salt, and pepper.

 - **Preparation**:

 - Preheat the oven to 375°F (190° C).

 - Scoop out the zucchini centres and combine with cooked turkey, quinoa, black beans, salsa and spices.

 - Fill the zucchini halves with the mixture and bake until they are cooked.

 - Nutritional Value: - Turkey provides lean protein, quinoa and beans provide fibre, and vegetables contain vitamins.

 - Cooking Time: 30 minutes

5. Mediterranean Chickpea Salad
Ingredients:

 - One can (15 ounces) of drained and washed chickpeas

Ingredients: 1 cup halved cherry tomatoes and 1 chopped cucumber.

- 1/4 cup finely chopped red onion.

- 1/2 cup crumbled feta cheese.

- Klamath olives, chopped

- Two teaspoons of olive oil.

- Add lemon juice, oregano, salt, and pepper to taste.

Preparation

- In a bowl, combine the chickpeas, tomatoes, cucumber, red onion, feta, and olives.

- Drizzle with olive oil, then add the lemon juice, oregano, salt, and pepper. Toss lightly.

- Nutritional Value: - Chickpeas and feta provide protein, olive oil contains healthy fats, and vegetables include antioxidants.

- Cook Time:

- 15 minutes (with canned chickpeas)

6. Veggie and Tofu Stir-Fry with Brown Rice

Ingredients:

- 1 cup cubed firm tofu, stir-fry vegetables (broccoli, carrots, bell peppers),
- 1 cup cooked brown rice
- 2 teaspoons low-sodium soy sauce.
- One tablespoon of sesame oil.
- 1 teaspoon of minced garlic.

- Preparation:

- In a wok or skillet, cook tofu and mixed vegetables in sesame oil with garlic.

- Stir in the cooked brown rice and soy sauce, cooking until well heated.

- Nutritive Value:

- Tofu provides plant-based protein, while brown rice and vegetables provide fibre and sesame oil provides healthy fats.

- Cook Time:

- Twenty minutes.

7. Lentil and Vegetable Soup

Ingredients:

- 1 cup rinsed and drained lentils.
- Mixed veggies (carrots, celery, and onions).
- 4 cups vegetable broth and 1 can of chopped tomatoes (14 ounces).
- One teaspoon of cumin, paprika, salt, and pepper

- **Preparation**:

- Sauté vegetables in a pot until tender. Combine lentils, broth, tomatoes, and spices.

- Simmer until the lentils are tender and the flavours blend.

- Nutritional Value: - Lentils provide protein, vegetables provide vitamins, and this is a low-calorie, high-fibre meal alternative.

- Cooking Time: 30 minutes

8. Chicken and Vegetable Quinoa Bowl

Ingredients:

- Four ounces of grilled chicken, sliced

- 1 cup cooked quinoa - Assorted vegetables (zucchini, bell peppers, cherry tomatoes)

- Two tablespoons balsamic vinaigrette.

- Fresh basil or parsley as garnish

- **Preparation**:

- Place sliced grilled chicken, cooked quinoa, and sautéed vegetables in a bowl.

- Drizzle with balsamic vinaigrette and sprinkle with fresh herbs.

- Nutritional Value: - Chicken provides lean protein, quinoa and vegetables provide fibre, and herbs include antioxidants.

- Cook Time:

- 20 minutes (including the quinoa boiling time).

9. Sweet Potato and Black Bean Quesadilla

Ingredients:

- Peel and shred one big sweet potato.
- Drain and rinse one can (15 ounces) of black beans.
- Whole-grain tortillas.

- 1 cup shredded cheese (either cheddar or Mexican blend)
- 1 teaspoon of cumin, chilli powder, salt, and pepper.

- Preparation:

- Cook grated sweet potatoes with black beans with seasonings until soft.

- Make quesadillas using the Ingredients, cheese, and whole grain tortillas. Cook until the cheese melts.

- Nutritive Value:

- Sweet potatoes with black beans provide fibre, beans provide protein, and tortillas contain nutritious grains.

- Cook Time:

- Twenty minutes.

10. Tuna and White Bean Salad

Ingredients:

- 1 can (5 oz) tuna, drained

- One can (15 ounces) of white beans, drained and rinsed

- Cherry tomatoes halved

Finely cut red onion and add 2 tablespoons olive oil.

- Add lemon juice, parsley, salt, and pepper to taste. - Prepare:

- Combine the tuna, white beans, tomatoes, and red onion in a bowl.

- Drizzle with olive oil, then add the lemon juice, parsley, salt, and pepper. Toss lightly.

- Nutritive Value:

- Tuna and beans provide protein, olive oil provide healthy fats, and vegetables contain vitamins.

- Cook Time: -10 minutes

DINNER

1. Baked lemon herb salmon

Ingredients:

- Two salmon fillets, 6 ounces each.

- one lemon, sliced

- Two teaspoons of olive oil.

- Fresh herbs (dill, parsley)

- Add salt and pepper to taste.

- **Preparation**:

- Preheat the oven to 400 °F (200°C).

  - Arrange the salmon fillets on a baking sheet, then top with lemon slices and herbs.

  - Drizzle with olive oil, season with salt and pepper, and bake until the salmon is thoroughly done.

  - Nutritive Value:

- Salmon provides omega-3 fatty acids, olive oil has healthful fats, and lemon contains vitamin C.

- Cooking time: 15 minutes.

2. Vegetarian quinoa-stuffed bell peppers

Ingredients:

- 4 halved bell peppers

- 1 cup cooked quinoa

- 1 can (15 ounces) of drained and rinsed black beans

- Corn kernels, cherry tomatoes and red onion, diced

- 1 teaspoon of cumin, chilli powder, salt, and pepper.

- **Preparation**:

- Preheat the oven to 375°F (190° C).

- Combine the quinoa, black beans, corn, tomatoes, red onion and spices.

- Stuff bell pepper halves with the mixture and bake until they are soft.

- Nutritional Value: Contains protein from black beans, fibre from quinoa and veggies, and vitamins from tomatoes.

- Cooking Time: 30 minutes

3. Grilled Chicken and Asparagus Salad

Ingredients:

- Two boneless, skinless chicken breasts.

- One bunch of trimmed asparagus

- Mixed salad greens.

- Cherry tomatoes halved

- Balsamic Vinaigrette

- Add salt and pepper to taste - **Preparation**:

- Grill the chicken breasts and asparagus until done.

- Slice the chicken and put it in a salad with mixed greens, asparagus, and tomatoes.

- Drizzle with balsamic vinaigrette, then season with salt and pepper.

- Nutritive Value:

- Chicken provides lean protein, vegetables contain fibre, and tomatoes contain antioxidants.

- Cook Time:

- Twenty minutes.

4. Spaghetti Squash with Turkey Bolognese

Ingredients:

1 medium spaghetti squash

1 pound of turkey

1 can (14 ounces) crushed tomatoes.

Dice one onion and mince two garlic cloves.

- Add Italian herbs, salt, and pepper to taste. - **Prepare:**

- Preheat the oven to 375°F (190° C).

- Cut spaghetti squash in half, remove the seeds, and bake until soft.

- Cook ground turkey in a skillet with onion, garlic, crushed tomatoes, and seasonings.

- Scrape spaghetti squash with a fork, then top with turkey Bolognese.

- Nutritional Value: - Turkey provides lean protein, tomatoes include vitamins, and spaghetti squash is a low-carb option.

- Cooking time: 45 minutes.

5. Shrimp and Vegetable Stir-Fry

Ingredients:

- 1 pound of peeled and deveined shrimp - Mixed stir-fry vegetables (broccoli, bell peppers, and snap peas)

- Two tablespoons of low-sodium soy sauce

- One tablespoon of sesame oil.

1 teaspoon grated ginger and 2 minced garlic cloves.

- **Preparation**:

- In a wok or skillet, cook prawns and mixed veggies in sesame oil with ginger and garlic.

- Add the soy sauce and simmer until the prawns are pink and the vegetables are soft.

- Nutritive Value:

- Shrimp provide protein, vegetables provide fibre, and sesame oil provides healthful fat.

- Cooking time: 15 minutes.

6. Stuffed Portobello Mushrooms with Quinoa and Spinach

Ingredients:

- 4 large Portobello mushrooms, cleaned and stemmed
- 1 cup cooked quinoa
- 1 cup chopped fresh spinach - 1/2 cup crumbled feta cheese
- Two teaspoons of olive oil.
- Add salt and pepper to taste.

- **Preparation**:

- Preheat the oven to 375°F (190° C).

- Combine the quinoa, spinach, feta, olive oil, salt, and pepper.

- Stuff Portobello mushrooms with the mixture and bake until they are soft.

- Nutritive Value:

    - Quinoa provides protein, spinach contains iron, and feta contains calcium.

- Cooking Time: 25 minutes.

7. Lemon Garlic Baked Cod

Ingredients:

- 4 cod fillets, 6 ounces each.

  - Zest and juice from 1 lemon

  - Two teaspoons of olive oil.

  - 2 garlic cloves, minced

  - Fresh parsley, chopped.

  - Add salt and pepper to taste

Preparation:

  - Preheat the oven to 400 °F (200°C).

  - Arrange cod fillets on a baking sheet.

- Combine the lemon zest, juice, olive oil, garlic, parsley, salt, and pepper. Pour over cod.

- Bake until the cod is flaky and cooked thoroughly.

- Nutritive Value:

- Cod provides lean protein, olive oil contains omega-3, and lemon contains vitamin C.

- Cook Time:

- 15 Minutes

8. Eggplant and Chickpea Curry

Ingredients:

- One large aubergine, diced

- One can (15 ounces) of drained and washed chickpeas

- One can of chopped tomatoes (14 ounces)

- 1 onion, diced

- 2 garlic cloves, minced

- One can of coconut milk (14 ounces)

- Two teaspoons of curry powder, turmeric, salt, and pepper.

- **Preparation**:

- In a pot, cook the aubergine, chickpeas, onions and garlic until tender.

- Combine diced tomatoes, coconut milk, and spices.

- Simmer until the flavours blend.

- Nutritional Value: - Chickpeas provide protein, eggplant contains fibre, and spices have anti-inflammatory qualities.

- Cooking Time: 30 minutes

9. Turkey and Vegetable Skewers

Ingredients:

1 pound ground turkey and cherry tomatoes.

- Bell peppers sliced into bits

Red onion, chopped into bits.

Olive oil, lemon juice, garlic, oregano, salt, and pepper.

- **Preparation**:

- Preheat the grill or grill pan.

- Combine the ground turkey with olive oil, lemon juice, garlic, oregano, salt, and pepper.

- Thread turkey and vegetable chunks on skewers and grill until done.

- Nutritional Value: - Turkey provides lean protein, vegetables provide vitamins, and grilling is a low-fat alternative.

- Cook Time: Twenty minutes.

10. Vegetarian Lentil and Sweet Potato Curry

Ingredients:

- 1 cup dried lentils, rinsed and drained

Ingredients: 2 peeled and diced sweet potatoes and 1 can (14 ounces) diced tomatoes.

- One can (14 ounces). Coconut Milk

Dice one onion and mince two garlic cloves.

- Two teaspoons of curry powder, cumin, salt, and pepper.

- **Preparation**:

- In a pot, add the lentils, sweet potatoes, tomatoes, coconut milk, onions, garlic, and spices.

- Simmer until the lentils and sweet potatoes are soft.

- Nutritional Value: - Lentils provide protein, sweet potatoes contain vitamins, and spices have anti-inflammatory effects.

- Cooking time: - 40 minutes

DESSERT

1. Greek Yoghurt Parfait with Berries

Ingredients:

- One cup of Greek yoghurt.

- Add 1/2 cup mixed berries (strawberries, blueberries, raspberries) and 2 tbsp granola.

Ingredients: - 1 teaspoon honey - **Preparation**:

- In a glass or dish, combine the Greek yoghurt, mixed berries, and granola.

- Drizzle the honey on top.

- Nutritive Value:

- Greek yoghurt provides protein, berries have antioxidants, and granola contains fibre.

- **Preparation** Time: 5 minutes.

2. Dark Chocolate Covered Strawberries

Ingredients

- Wash and dry 1 cup strawberries. - Melt 3 ounces of dark chocolate.

- **Preparation**: Dip each strawberry in melted dark chocolate, covering half.

- Place on parchment paper and let cool until the chocolate hardens.

- Nutritive Value:

- Dark chocolate contains antioxidants, while strawberries provide vitamins.

- **Preparation** time: - 15 minutes

3. Baked cinnamon apple chips

Ingredients:

- Two finely sliced apples - One teaspoon cinnamon

- One tablespoon of honey (optional).

- **Preparation**:

- Preheat the oven to 225°F (110° C).

- Toss apple slices with cinnamon and honey, if using.

- Place on a baking sheet and bake until crispy.

- Nutritive Value:

- Apples provide fibre, cinnamon contains antioxidants, and there is natural sweetness.

- Cooking time: 2 hours.

4. Chia Seed Pudding with Mango

Ingredients:

- Three tablespoons of chia seeds

- One cup almond milk.

Add 1/2 teaspoon vanilla extract and 1/2 cup cubed mango.

- **Preparation**:

- Combine chia seeds, almond milk, and vanilla extract in a jar.

- Refrigerate overnight, then top with diced mango before serving.

- Nutritional Value: - Chia seeds provide omega-3 fatty acids and mango contains vitamins.

- **Preparation** Time: - 5 minutes, plus overnight refrigeration.

5. Trail Mix with Nuts and Dried Fruits

Ingredients:

-1/2 cup almonds

-1/4 cup walnuts

- 1/4 cup dried cranberries.

-1/4 cup pumpkin seeds

- **Preparation**:

- Combine all items in a bowl.

- Divide into **Snack**-sized bags for convenience.

Nutritional Value: - Nuts provide healthy fats and protein, while dried fruits contain antioxidants.

- Prep Time:

- Five minutes.

6. Cacao Nib and Date Energy bar

Ingredients:

- One cup of pitted dates

-1/2 cup almonds

Ingredients: 1/4 cup cacao nibs, 1/4 cup shredded coconut.

- **Preparation**:

- In a food processor, combine dates, almonds, cacao nibs, and shredded coconut. Process until a sticky dough forms.

- Press the mixture into a lined pan and chill until stiff. Cut into bars.

- Nutritive Value:

- Dates provide fibre, while almonds and cacao nibs contain healthful fats.

- **Preparation** Time: - 15 minutes (including chilling time)

7. Blueberry Oat Muffins

Ingredients:

Ingredients: 1 cup rolled oats, 1 cup milk.

- One cup whole wheat flour.

- 1/4 cup melted coconut oil.

-1/4 cup honey

- 1 egg - 1 tbsp baking powder

-1/2 teaspoon cinnamon

- 1 cup blueberries, fresh or frozen.

- **Preparation**:

- Preheat the oven to 375° Fahrenheit (190° Celsius). Line the muffin tray with liners.

- In a bowl, soak the oats in milk for 10 minutes.

- Combine the flour, melted coconut oil, honey, egg, baking powder, and cinnamon. Fold in blueberries.

- Spoon the batter into the muffin cups and bake until a toothpick comes clean.

- Nutritional Value: - Oats provide fibre, blueberries contain antioxidants, and honey adds natural sweetness.

- Baking Time:

- Twenty minutes.

8. Avocado Chocolate Mousse

Ingredients:

- two ripe avocados.

- 1/4 cup unsweetened cocoa powder.

- 1/4 cup honey or maple syrup.

- One teaspoon vanilla extract.

- One pinch of salt.

- **Preparation**:

- Blend avocados, cocoa powder, honey or maple syrup, vanilla extract, and salt until smooth.

- Refrigerate for at least 30 minutes before serving.

- Nutritional value: - Avocados provide healthy fats, chocolate contains antioxidants, and honey or maple syrup adds natural sweetness.

- **Preparation** time: 10 minutes, including cooling time.

9. Strawberry Banana Ice Cream

Ingredients:

- 2 cups frozen strawberries - 2 ripe bananas (sliced and frozen)

Add 1/4 cup almond milk and 1 teaspoon honey (optional).

- **Preparation**:

- Blend frozen strawberries, banana slices, almond milk, and honey until smooth.

- Serve immediately for a tasty strawberry banana ice cream.

- Nutritive Value:

- Strawberries have vitamins, bananas contain potassium, and it is naturally sweet.

- **Preparation** Time: 5 minutes.

10. Almond Joy Energy Bites

Ingredients:

1/2 cup almond butter.

1 cup rolled oats

1/4 cup honey

1/4 cup shredded coconut.

1/4 cup dark chocolate chips.

Preparation:

- Combine the rolled oats, almond butter, honey, shredded coconut, and dark chocolate chips in a bowl.

- Form into bite-size balls and chill until solid.

- Nutritive Value:

- Oats provide fibre, almond butter and coconut include healthy fats, while dark chocolate has antioxidants.

- Prep Time: - 15 minutes, plus chilling time.

MEAL PLANNING

Day 1

- ✔ **Breakfast::** Greek Yoghurt Parfait with Berries (1 cup Greek yoghurt, 1/2 cup mixed berries, and 2 tbsp granola
- ✔ **Lunch**: Quinoa Salad with Grilled Chicken (1 cup cooked quinoa, 4 ounces grilled chicken, cherry tomatoes, cucumber, and feta cheese.
- ✔ **Snack**: Trail mix (almonds, walnuts, dried cranberries, pumpkin seeds)
- ✔ **Dinner**: Baked Lemon Herb Salmon (2 salmon fillets, lemon slices, olive oil, herbs) with steamed asparagus.

Day 2

- ✔ **Breakfast::** Chia Seed Pudding with Mango (3 tablespoons chia seeds, 1 cup almond milk, 1/2 teaspoon vanilla extract, and 1/2 cup sliced mango)

✔ **Lunch**: Lentil and Vegetable Soup (1 cup lentils, mixed veggies, vegetable broth, chopped tomatoes)

✔ **Snack**: Banana and Walnut Muffin (one muffin)

✔ **Dinner**: Stuffed Portobello Mushrooms with Quinoa and Spinach (4 large portobello mushrooms, quinoa, fresh spinach, feta cheese)

Day 3

✔ **Breakfast::** Berry Smoothie Bowl (1 cup mixed berries, 1/2 banana, 1/2 cup Greek yoghurt, 1/4 cup granola.

✔ **Lunch**: Chicken and Vegetable Quinoa Bowl (4 oz grilled chicken, 1 cup cooked quinoa, mixed vegetables, balsamic vinaigrette).

✔ **Snack**: Cacao Nib and Date Energy Bars (one bar)

✔ **Dinner**: Eggplant and Chickpea Curry (1 large eggplant, chickpeas, chopped tomatoes, coconut milk).

Day 4

✔ **Breakfast::** Oatmeal Raisin Energy Bites (1 cup rolled oats, 1/2 cup almond butter, 1/4 cup honey, 1/4 cup raisins.

✔ **Lunch**: Mediterranean Chickpea Salad (one can chickpeas, cherry tomatoes, cucumber, red onion, feta cheese, olives)

✔ **Snack**: Greek Yoghurt with Honey and Almonds (1 cup Greek yoghurt, drizzled with honey, handful of almonds)

✔ **Dinner**: Turkey and Quinoa Stuffed Zucchini (two zucchini, ground turkey, cooked quinoa, black beans, salsa)

Day 5

✔ **Breakfast::** Frozen banana bites (2 bananas, 1/4 cup peanut butter, and dark chocolate chips)

✔ **Lunch**: Veggie and Tofu Stir-Fry with Brown Rice (1 cup firm tofu, mixed stir-fried vegetables, and 1 cup cooked brown rice)

✔ **Snack**: Hummus and Veggie **Snack** Plate (half cup hummus, carrot sticks, cucumber slices, cherry tomatoes)

✔ **Dinner**: Grilled Chicken with Asparagus Salad (2 boneless, skinless chicken breasts, asparagus, mixed salad greens)

Day 6

- ✔ **Breakfast::** Blueberry Muffins (1 cup rolled oats, 1 cup milk, 1 cup whole wheat flour, coconut oil, honey, egg, baking powder, cinnamon, 1 cup blueberries).
- ✔ **Lunch**: Tuna and White Bean Salad (1 can tuna, one can white beans, cherry tomatoes, red onion, olive oil, lemon juice)
- ✔ **Snack**: Coconut and Almond Energy Balls (1 ball).
- ✔ **Dinner**: Shrimp and Vegetable Stir-Fry (1 pound shrimp, mixed stir-fry vegetables, low-sodium soy sauce, sesame oil)

Day 7

- ✔ **Breakfast::** Avocado Chocolate Mousse (2 ripe avocados, 1/4 cup unsweetened cocoa powder, 1/4 cup honey or maple syrup, 1 teaspoon vanilla extract.

- ✔ **Lunch**: Sweet Potato and Black Bean Quesadilla (1 large sweet potato, one can black beans, whole grain tortillas, cumin, and chilli powder)

- ✔ **Snack**: Berry Smoothie with Spinach (1 cup mixed berries, 1 cup spinach, 1/2 banana, and 1/2 cup almond milk).

- ✔ **Dinner**: Vegetable and Lentil Curry (Mixed veggies, 1 cup dried lentils, diced tomatoes, coconut milk, curry powder)

Day 8

- **Breakfast::** Strawberry Banana Ice Cream (2 cups frozen strawberries, 2 ripe bananas, 1/4 cup almond milk, 1 teaspoon honey)

- **Lunch**: Greek Salad with Grilled Chicken (4 ounces grilled chicken, mixed greens, cherry tomatoes, cucumber, olives, feta cheese).

- **Snack**: Almond Joy Energy Bites (1 cup rolled oats, 1/2 cup almond butter, 1/4 cup honey, 1/4 cup shredded coconut, 1/4 cup dark chocolate chips)

- **Dinner**: Baked Cod with Lemon Garlic Sauce (4 cod fillets, lemon zest and juice, olive oil, garlic, parsley)

Day 9

✔ **Breakfast::** Cucumber and Avocado Salsa (1 cucumber, one avocado, 1/4 cup red onion, 1/4 cup cilantro, lime juice)

- ✔ **Lunch**: Quinoa and Vegetable Wrap (one cup cooked quinoa, mixed grilled vegetables, whole grain wrap)
- ✔ **Snack**: Frozen Yoghurt Bark with Nuts and Berries. (1 cup Greek yoghurt, 1 tablespoon honey, 1/4 cup mixed nuts, 1/4 cup mixed berries).
- ✔ **Dinner**: Chickpea and Spinach Stew (one can chickpeas, fresh spinach, chopped tomatoes, vegetable broth, spices)

Day 10

- ✔ **Breakfast::** Pumpkin Chia Seed Pudding (1/2 cup canned pumpkin puree, 3 tablespoons chia seeds, 1 cup almond milk, 1/2 teaspoon pumpkin spice, and 1 tablespoon maple syrup
- ✔ **Lunch**: Caprese Quinoa Salad (1 cup cooked quinoa, cherry tomatoes, fresh

mozzarella, basil, and balsamic sauce).

- ✔ **Snack**: Dark Chocolate Covered Strawberries (1 cup strawberries; 3 ounces dark chocolate)
- ✔ **Dinner**: Vegetarian Lentil and Sweet Potato Curry (1 cup dry lentils, 2 sweet potatoes, diced tomatoes, coconut milk, curry powder)

Day 11

- ✔ **Breakfast::** Trail mix with nuts and dried fruits (almonds, walnuts, dried cranberries, and pumpkin seeds).
- ✔ **Lunch**: Spinach and Feta Stuffed Chicken Breast (2 boneless skinless chicken breasts, fresh spinach, and feta cheese)

✔ **Snack**: Apple and Almond Butter Slices (1 apple + 2 tbsp almond butter)

✔ **Dinner**: Quinoa-Stuffed Bell Peppers (4 bell peppers, 1 cup cooked quinoa, one can black beans, corn, tomatoes, cumin, chilli powder)

Day 12

✔ **Breakfast::** Coconut Yoghurt Parfait with Tropical Fruits (1 cup coconut yoghurt, pineapple chunks, mango slices, and shredded coconut)

✔ **Lunch**: Mediterranean Hummus Wrap (whole grain wrap with hummus, cucumber, cherry tomatoes, olives, and feta cheese)

✔ **Snack**: Greek Yoghurt and Berry Popsicle (1 cup Greek yoghurt and mixed berries)

✔ **Dinner**: Salmon and Vegetable Skewers (2 salmon fillets, cherry tomatoes, bell peppers, and red onion).

Day 13

✔ **Breakfast::** Berry and Spinach Smoothie (1 cup mixed berries, 1 cup spinach, 1/2 banana, and 1/2 cup almond milk).

✔ **Lunch**: Quinoa and Black Bean Bowl (1 cup cooked quinoa, one can black beans, corn, avocado and salsa)

✔ **Snack**: Apple and Cheese Slices (1 apple + 1 ounce cheese)

✔ **Dinner**: Grilled Veggie and Chickpea Salad (Mixed grilled vegetables, one can chickpeas, feta cheese, balsamic vinaigrette).

Day 14

- ✔ **Breakfast::** Acai Bowl with Granola and Berries (1/2 cup granola, mixed berries)

- ✔ **Lunch**: Turkey and Vegetable Skewers (1 pound of turkey, cherry tomatoes, bell peppers, red onion, olive oil, lemon juice, garlic, oregano).

- ✔ **Snack**: Pumpkin Spice Protein Smoothie (1/2 cup canned pumpkin puree, 1 scoop protein powder, almond milk, and pumpkin spice).

- ✔ **Dinner**: Spaghetti Squash with Turkey Bolognese (1 medium-sized spaghetti squash, 1 pound ground turkey, 1 can crushed tomatoes, onion, garlic, Italian herbs)

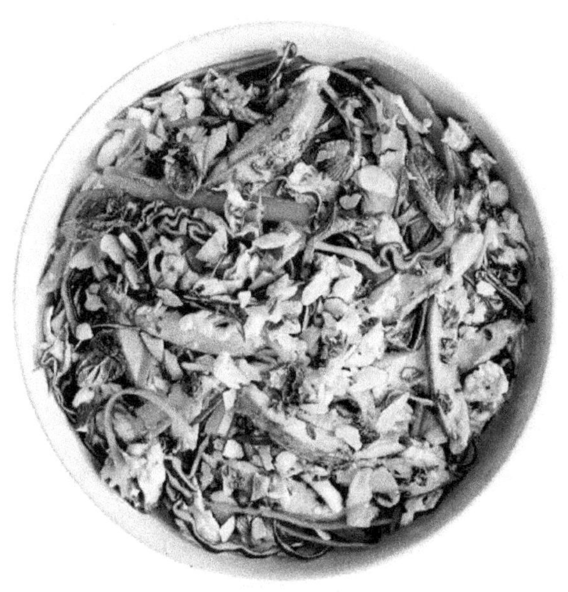

CONCLUSION

To summarise, this Breast Cancer Disease Cookbook for Newly Diagnosed Individuals is more than just a collection of dishes; it is a guide to adopting a healthy lifestyle. The carefully created meal plans and different recipes not only meet the nutritional demands of women confronting a breast cancer diagnosis, but also highlight the joy of eating healthy and delectable foods. This cookbook strives to empower people to make positive choices for their health by incorporating nutrient-rich **Ingredients**, emphasising anti-inflammatory characteristics, and advocating for a well-balanced diet.

Remember, this journey is about more than simply the food on your plate; it is also about the empowerment it brings into your life. Each dish is a step towards reclaiming control and embracing a healthy lifestyle. As you embark on this culinary adventure, may you find strength, comfort, and a new feeling of life?

Portion sizes can be adjusted to meet individual nutritional needs and preferences. When developing a specific meal plan, it is critical to speak with a healthcare professional or nutritionist, particularly for people dealing with health issues such as breast cancer.

6 WEEK MEAL PLANNER

MEAL PLANNER

MONDAY

BREAKFAST _______________________

LUNCH _______________________

DINNER _______________________

TUESDAY

BREAKFAST _______________________

LUNCH _______________________

DINNER _______________________

WEDNESDAY

BREAKFAST _______________________

LUNCH _______________________

DINNER _______________________

THURSDAY

BREAKFAST _______________________

LUNCH _______________________

DINNER _______________________

FRIDAY

BREAKFAST _______________________

LUNCH _______________________

DINNER _______________________

SATURDAY

BREAKFAST _______________________

LUNCH _______________________

DINNER _______________________

SUNDAY

BREAKFAST _______________________

LUNCH _______________________

DINNER _______________________

NOTE:

SHOPPING LIST

____

____

____

____

____

____

____

____

MEAL PLANNER

MONDAY

BREAKFAST _______________________

LUNCH _______________________

DINNER _______________________

TUESDAY

BREAKFAST _______________________

LUNCH _______________________

DINNER _______________________

WEDNESDAY

BREAKFAST _______________________

LUNCH _______________________

DINNER _______________________

THURSDAY

BREAKFAST _______________________

LUNCH _______________________

DINNER _______________________

FRIDAY

BREAKFAST _______________________

LUNCH _______________________

DINNER _______________________

SATURDAY

BREAKFAST _______________________

LUNCH _______________________

DINNER _______________________

SUNDAY

BREAKFAST _______________________

LUNCH _______________________

DINNER _______________________

NOTE:

SHOPPING LIST

____

____

____

____

____

____

____

MEAL PLANNER

MONDAY
BREAKFAST _________________

LUNCH _________________

DINNER _________________

TUESDAY
BREAKFAST _________________

LUNCH _________________

DINNER _________________

WEDNESDAY
BREAKFAST _________________

LUNCH _________________

DINNER _________________

THURSDAY
BREAKFAST _________________

LUNCH _________________

DINNER _________________

FRIDAY
BREAKFAST _________________

LUNCH _________________

DINNER _________________

SATURDAY
BREAKFAST _________________

LUNCH _________________

DINNER _________________

SUNDAY
BREAKFAST _________________

LUNCH _________________

DINNER _________________

NOTE:

SHOPPING LIST
____

____

____

____

____

____

____

MEAL PLANNER

<table>
<tr><td>

MONDAY

BREAKFAST ___________________

LUNCH ___________________

DINNER ___________________

</td><td>

TUESDAY

BREAKFAST ___________________

LUNCH ___________________

DINNER ___________________

</td></tr>
<tr><td>

WEDNESDAY

BREAKFAST ___________________

LUNCH ___________________

DINNER ___________________

</td><td>

THURSDAY

BREAKFAST ___________________

LUNCH ___________________

DINNER ___________________

</td></tr>
<tr><td>

FRIDAY

BREAKFAST ___________________

LUNCH ___________________

DINNER ___________________

</td><td>

SATURDAY

BREAKFAST ___________________

LUNCH ___________________

DINNER ___________________

</td></tr>
<tr><td>

SUNDAY

BREAKFAST ___________________

LUNCH ___________________

DINNER ___________________

NOTE:

</td><td>

SHOPPING LIST

____

____

____

____

____

____

____

</td></tr>
</table>

MEAL PLANNER

MONDAY

BREAKFAST _______________________

LUNCH _______________________

DINNER _______________________

TUESDAY

BREAKFAST _______________________

LUNCH _______________________

DINNER _______________________

WEDNESDAY

BREAKFAST _______________________

LUNCH _______________________

DINNER _______________________

THURSDAY

BREAKFAST _______________________

LUNCH _______________________

DINNER _______________________

FRIDAY

BREAKFAST _______________________

LUNCH _______________________

DINNER _______________________

SATURDAY

BREAKFAST _______________________

LUNCH _______________________

DINNER _______________________

SUNDAY

BREAKFAST _______________________

LUNCH _______________________

DINNER _______________________

NOTE:

SHOPPING LIST

____

____

____

____

____

____

____

MEAL PLANNER

BREAKFAST ___________________

LUNCH ___________________

DINNER ___________________

BREAKFAST ___________________

LUNCH ___________________

DINNER___________________

BREAKFAST ___________________

LUNCH ___________________

DINNER ___________________

BREAKFAST ___________________

LUNCH ___________________

DINNER ___________________

BREAKFAST ___________________

LUNCH ___________________

DINNER___________________

BREAKFAST ___________________

LUNCH ___________________

DINNER ___________________

BREAKFAST ___________________
LUNCH ___________________
DINNER ___________________

NOTE:

____
____
____
____
____
____
____

www.ingramcontent.com/pod-product-compliance
Lightning Source LLC
Chambersburg PA
CBHW050834260726

48660CB00006B/2232